Weight Loss

An Effective Diet Plan For Losing Weight In 2 Weeks

Table of contents

Introduction

There a hundreds of different diets on the market, many of which promise some magical formula to making you lose weight. Some advise cutting out entire food groups, not 'combining' certain foods, not eating at certain times of the day, or using smaller plates and chewing your food a regulation number of times. Many of them also promise to be 'easy' or that you will never experience hunger.

ALL diets work by making the body burn more calories than it consumes – every single "rule" that these diets promote is simply a way to encourage you to eat fewer calories. It is not realistic to expect to never feel hungry – hunger is your body's signal that it needs more calories. You can fill your stomach with low-calorie, high bulk foods to encourage a feeling of 'fullness' but you must be prepared to also experience hunger.

Learning to differentiate true hunger from a specific craving is very useful. You should learn to eat only when you are truly hungry, and stop eating once you are full. Eating if you are not truly hungry is a sure-fire way to eat not only too much food, but the wrong kinds of foods. If you are not hungry, then the temptation will be to eat high-sugar, high "reward" food so that your body feels satisfied. If you are sating true hunger, then your food will taste better and you will not require "treat" foods that are high in sugar and salt.

Hunger which is regularly satisfied should not be uncomfortable. Plan your meals in advance, so that you know that your hunger will only last a certain length of time, and look forward to what you are going to eat. This way, you have no reason to feel guilty about what you have eaten.

In the West, we live in surrounded by food and advertisements for food, each one attempting to persuade us to consume their product over the others. Millions of pounds every year is spent so that we will want new, more enjoyable, more elaborate foods. We are also constantly bombarded with information about the obesity epidemic; these two messages standing side by side, both lecturing us about what we should and should not be eating. Add to this the Media's obsession with so-called super foods, organic foods, and the methods by which our food is grown and processed, and it is no wonder that many people find the whole question of what and how much to eat overwhelming. We are a culture which fetishises this basic human drive – to feed ourselves.

You can take back control over what you eat. Try to be aware of what is motivating you each time you make a food choice – is it hunger, guilt, tiredness or even a sense of obligation? As children, we were often told to 'eat up; to please a parent , and many people carry this feeling of eating being something that pleases others into adulthood with them. Be aware of your own particular food triggers to help you make better choices.

Chapter 1 – Breakfast

There are two main approaches to breakfast that most dieters take. The first is to skip it entirely, in the belief that it will 'get the day off to a good start'. The second is to regard breakfast as so essential that anything eaten in the mornings is a 'free go'. There are problems with both these scenarios:

1) "I will skip breakfast entirely to save calories"

This, in itself, is not necessarily a bad strategy. If you generally do not feel like eating anything in the morning, then there is no point forcing yourself to do so. Many traditional breakfast foods are not especially healthy; cereals are often terrifyingly high in sugar and a slice of whole meal toast is unlikely to keep you from being hungry before lunchtime.

The danger of this strategy is that it can lead to snacking later on. If you skip breakfast at 7am but pick up a croissant on your way to work, or end up eating several biscuits at 11 o'clock, this method clearly does not work *for you*. If you skip breakfast and find yourself hungry later, make sure you snack on something from the healthy list below. Remember, it is total calories consumed that matter, not when you ate them.

2) "I will eat a large breakfast, since it is the most important meal of the day. This will give me plenty of time to burn off the extra calories, and it will encourage my metabolism to work faster, thus making the calories matter less"

The human metabolism is extremely complex, and varies from person to person. You cannot tinker around with it to reset it at a higher rate simply by eating a larger breakfast – the only things that can genuinely alter your metabolism are drugs, which come with dangerous side effects. Again, it is total calories that matter. If you eat a large breakfast which means that you are able to eat a smaller lunch, then this is a good strategy *for you*. If you eat a large breakfast, but still find yourself snacking by 11am, you should save the calories from breakfast to eat later in the day.

Breakfast Recipes:

Time can be limited in the morning. The important thing is to try to have some protein (which will give you a feeling of fullness) and avoid too much refined sugar, as many people find this quickly leaves them feeling hungry again.

Poached Eggs with Asparagus:

You will need:

2 large free range eggs

5 – 6 asparagus spears

Method:

Trim the woody ends from the asparagus spears. Bring a pan of salted water to the boil, and cook the spears until the ends soften. Remove and cover to keep warm.

Bring the water to a gentle simmer. Swirl the water (it will be slightly green) and crack the eggs into the centre of the whirlpool you have just created. For runny yolks, cook for three to four minutes, then remove with a slotted spoon. Dab the eggs gently with kitchen paper to remove the excess water, and serve immediately with the asparagus.

Breakfast Tortilla:

This is the ideal dish to prepare in advance. Just grab a wedge from the fridge to eat before you leave for work.

You will need:

6 free range eggs

1 small onion, sliced

1 red pepper, deseeded and sliced (you could also use pre-prepared bottled peppers)

Half a small tin of sweetcorn

A handful of fresh spinach leaves, washed

150g of grated strong cheddar

Salt and pepper

Sliced red chili (optional)

Fresh herbs such as parsley or basil

Method:

Cook the onion in a non-stick pan with a little olive oil for a few minutes until it begins to soften, then add the pepper and continue to cook. Stir through the sweetcorn. In a bowl, beat together the eggs and season well. Drop in the spinach to the pan and stir as it wilts – this will only take a couple of seconds. Pour in the beaten eggs and stir, scraping the bottom of the pan to combine the cooked egg. Add the herbs, if using.

Once the egg has thickened, turn the heat right down and sprinkle over the grated cheese. Allow the pan to cook for a few more minutes, until the tortilla starts to lift away from the sides. Slide the pan under a hot grill to set the top and make the cheese bubble.

Once the tortilla is cooked in the centre, remove from the heat and cut into wedges. You can eat these hot or cold.

Melon and Parma Ham:

This classic canapé is also great for the mornings, combining as it does fruit with protein.

You will need:

Some ripe melon – choose one with firm flesh, such as honeydew or cantaloupe rather than watermelon

Six slices of parma ham

Method:

Cut the melon into thin slices, then wind the ham around each slice. Eat straight away.

Apple Nut Butter:

The ideal grab and run breakfast. Simply slice an apple and spread each piece with the nut butter of your choosing – peanut, cashew or almond.

Porridge:

You will need:

50g porridge oats

350ml of water or milk

A spoonful of Greek yoghurt

A drizzle of honey

Method:

Put the oats, a pinch of salt, and water/milk in a high-sided bowl and microwave on high for 2 ½ minutes. Stir, then microwave for a further 2 ½ minutes. Leave the oats to stand for 2 minutes, then pour over the yoghurt and honey and serve.

Scrambled Egg and Mushrooms:

2 large eggs

Salt and pepper

A handful of mushrooms – white, button, Portobello or chestnut.

Method:

Slice the mushrooms and sauté in a non-stick pan over a high heat to drive off the water. When they have cooked through, beat the eggs in a bowl and season well, then pour into the pan and stir as they cook. Once the egg is cooked to your liking, scoop onto a plate and eat immediately.

Beans on Toast:

The humble baked bean is high in salt, but is also a great source of protein and fibre.

You will need:

1 small slice of wholemeal bread

50g of baked beans

Method:

Microwave the beans on high for one minute, then stir and microwave again until they are heated through. Toast the bread and pour over the beans. For added flavour, add some hot sauce, such as Tabasco or Sriracha, to the beans.

Ham Omlette:

You will need:

2 free range eggs

1 slice of ham, chopped

Salt and pepper

Method:

Beat the eggs and season well. In a non-stick pan, scatter the ham pieces, then pour over the eggs. Wait a few seconds for the egg to start to set, then draw in the sides with a spatula and swirl the pan so that the uncooked egg runs onto the cooking surface. Turn down the heat and allow to cook until the centre is almost set (or to individual preference) and serve straight away.

Chapter 2 – Snacks

Snacks are important -- some people find it impossible to concentrate if they are waiting for lunch or dinner time. However, you should not feel that you 'have' to snack. Some diet regimes insist on you consuming "three meals and two snacks" a day and although many people enjoy this regularity, it is not a magic formula for losing weight. It is based on the idea that you must prevent your body from going into "starvation mode" which is a situation where it hoards calories and reduces your metabolism, thus making it harder to lose weight.

In reality, "starvation mode" (even if it exists) would not be triggered by not eating between 1pm and 7pm. You should snack if you find that you are too hungry to wait for your next meal, overeat at the next opportunity, or that you end up making bad food choices because you have become too hungry to resist. Think about the overall calories you are consuming in a day – if resisting having a snack of 100 calories means that you overeat by 250 calories at dinner, it is clearly better to have the snack.

Banana and Honey: Mash a ripe banana with a drizzle of honey and microwave for a few seconds to warm through. It may look like baby food, but it will taste deliciously sweet and is full of fibre to keep you feeling fuller for longer.

Edamame Beans: These are now often sold in pots as snacks, but you can also buy them frozen for a much lower price. Popping the beans out of their shells is time-consuming (meaning you eat fewer) and they are high in protein and fibre.

Raw Nuts: Choose unsalted, unroasted nuts, such as cashews, brazil nuts or pistachios. Nibble on them slowly, they contain important nutrients and vitamins, and the high protein and oil levels will help to keep you feeling full.

Fruit: Fruit is always a good choice for a snack, however, it does contain high levels of sugar. You should steer clear of grapes all together; it is far too easy to mindlessly consume half a bunch without noticing.

You should also be careful about fruit smoothies – although they boast about containing 'whole fruit' they have often had most of the fibre (in the form of skins and cores) removed, meaning that they are as sugary as a soda.

Choose fruits where you eat as much of the whole fruit as possible – berries, apples, and kiwis are all good choices.

Diet Hot Chocolate: It is often a good idea to steer clear of so-called diet products, as they often replace fat with sugar (never a good trade) or are full of artificial ingredients. However, at 60 calories, a mug of low-calorie hot chocolate can be an excellent sweet-fix, as well as taking time to drink, meaning that your body feels more satisfied. You can even add a sprinkling of mini marshmallows without raising the calorie content to over 100.

Smoked Salmon Rolls: A little more work, but these could almost be a lunch – for only 106 calories. Cut 50g of smoked salmon into four equal strips and spoon 5g of cream cheese onto one end of each strip. Roll the strips up and eat – you can also add a sprig of dill for extra flavour.

Popcorn: this is a great alternative to crisps – just steer clear of ones with toffee or butter toppings. You can make your own and season with chili or Worcestershire sauce.

Hard boiled eggs: Great to make in advance and bring from home, a hard boiled egg is roughly 100 calories of pure protein. There used to be a convention that you should only eat two eggs a week (due to concerns over cholesterol), but this has long since been discounted. Eggs are safe and healthy, and you can eat as many as you want to.

(There is also a long running myth that eating too many eggs will make you constipated. This is simply not true – the confusion has arisen from a misunderstanding of the word 'eggbound'. Being eggbound is a condition in which chickens are unable to lay eggs properly, not humans being unable to move their bowels.)

Chapter 3 – Lunch

If you work outside the home, try to avoid letting yourself get into a situation when you decide what you want for lunch *once you are already hungry*. This is a dangerous scenario: you will choose unhealthy, high-calorie options, and justify it to yourself as a one-off.

If you decide on or prepare your food for lunch in advance, not only will you make better decisions about what to eat, you will also enjoy your food more. If you know what you are having for lunch – say, roasted vegetables with brown rice – then every time you feel hungry in the morning, your thoughts will turn to that. By the time you come to eat, it will seem like the only dish in the world that would satisfy you at that moment.

Your lunch choices will depend on the facilities available at your work. You may have access to microwaves, grills and even ovens, or you may just have a kettle and a toaster. Be careful if you do not have a fridge, or if the fridge is dirty and/or overstocked. You should not store cooked chicken or anything with raw egg (such as mayonnaise) unless you have access to a fridge that you are confident about.

Chickpea Pita Bread:

You will need:

1 whole-wheat pita

½ a cooked chicken breast

1 Tablespoon of chickpeas

1 Tablespoon of Greek yogurt

Fresh parsley and oregano (optional)

Method:

Toast the pita bread and split it open. Mix together the chick peas, yoghurt and herbs, and season. You can also add a little chopped fresh chilli for extra heat. Spread the mixture onto the pita and sprinkle over the chopped chicken breast.

Black Bean Wrap:

You will need:

1 whole-wheat wrap

1 Tablespoon of tinned black beans, drained and rinsed

¼ of one ripe avocado, sliced

2 spring onions, chopped

Hot sauce such as Sriracha or Tabasco (optional)

Method:

Warm the wrap and mash the avocado onto half of it. Mix together the remaining ingredients and roll up the wrap. You can also add salad leaves if you wish.

Salmon Caesar Salad Wrap:

You will need:

1 whole-wheat pita

75g of canned salmon

2 tablespoons of low calorie Caesar salad dressing

1 tablespoon of grated parmesan cheese

A handful of fresh spinach leaves

Method:

Drain the canned salmon (look for one which has been canned in spring water, not oil) and spread over half of the wrap. Mix together the spinach, dressing and parmesan, then add to the wrap and roll up.

Puy Lentil Salad with Poached Eggs:

You will need:

1 heaped tablespoon of canned puy lentils

A handful of fresh spinach

A small clove of garlic, chopped

2 large eggs

¼ of a ripe avocado

1 ripe tomato, sliced

Method:

Heat a pan with a little olive oil. Saute the garlic until it softens, stirring continuously to prevent it from burning, then add the spinach. When the spinach wilts, add the lentils and stir until heated through.

Meanwhile, bring a pan of salted water to the boil, swirl to make a whirlpool and drop in two eggs. Poach for three minutes, then remove from the water and dry on kitchen paper.

Chop the tomato and avocado, remove the lentils from the heat in and stir through. Serve with the poached eggs on top of the lentils and season to taste.

Curried Egg Salad:

2 hard boiled eggs

1 Tablespoon of Greek yoghurt

1 Teaspoon of hot curry powder

1 Large poppadom

Method:

Chop the eggs and mix with the yoghurt and curry powder. Scoop up with shards of the poppadom.

Roasted Beetroot and Goat's Cheese Salad:

You will need:

2 roasted baby beets, cut into wedges

2 handfuls of young leaf salad, such as Lamb's lettuce or spinach

50g crumbled goat's cheese

Olive oil and balsamic vinegar to dress

Method:

Whisk together the oil and vinegar with a little salt and pepper, and pour over the leaves. Add the beetroot and sprinkle over the goat's cheese.

Home -Made Homous With Pitta

You will need:

1 x 400g canned chick peas

2 Tablespoons of extra virgin olive oil

Salt and pepper

The juice of half a lemon

A little warm water

1 Tablespoon of Tahini paste

1 wholewheat pita bread

Method:

Use a stick blender or food processor to combine all ingredients (apart from the pita bread) and blend until smooth. Toast the pita and use to scoop up the homous. This recipe makes two servings of homous – cover the leftovers and store in the fridge.

Chapter 4 – Dinners

Chili Tenderloin of Pork with Sweet Potato

You will need:

1 pork tenderloin, trimmed of excess fat and sinew

A little olive oil

1 teaspoon of hot chili powder (adjust to personal taste)

2 tablespoons of maple syrup

Salt and pepper

500g of sweet potatoes, peeled and grated

3 shallots, cut into rings

2 handfuls of baby spinach, washed and chopped

hot sauce such as Tabasco or Sriracha (optional)

Method:

Preheat oven to 180 degrees. Rub the pork a little oil and chilli powder, and season well. Seal in an oven proof frying pan and then baste them with half of the maple syrup. Bake in the oven for 12 minutes, basting with the remaining syrup halfway through the cooking process. Remove from the oven when cooked through (pork can be served slightly rare in the middle, so cook it according to personal taste). Allow to rest.

Heat a little oil in a deep frying pan, and saute the shallots for a few minutes until softened, but do not allow to burn, Add the grated sweet potatoes and stir frequently for 10 minutes until the sweet potatoes are soft and beginning to colour slightly. Add the spinach and allow it to wilt.

Slice the pork and serve with a scoop of the potato hash.

White Fish with Cous Cous:

2 filets of firm white fish, such as cod or tilapia

1 lemon, half of it juiced, the other half cut into wedges for servings

1 Tablespoon of olive oil

2 cloves of garlic

Salt and pepper

150g cous cous

A small bunch of flat leafed parsley, chopped

2 tablespoons of sun-dried tomatoes, chopped (optional)

Method:

Mix together the olive oil, lemon juice, garlic, and seasoning. Marinade the fish fillets briefly, turning to coat thoroughly. Leave the fillets for ten minutes.

Cook the couscous according to the instructions on the package. Mix through the parsley and sun-dried tomatoes, if using.

Heat your grill to its highest setting. Place the fish fillets on an oiled sheet of tin foil and grill for a couple of minutes each side, depending on the thickness of the fillet. Serve with a scoop of cous cous and a wedge of fresh lemon.

Scallops and Sugar Snap Peas:

You Will Need:

150g of cous cous

3 tablespoons of olive oil

12 scallops, roes removed

salt and pepper

350g sugar snap peas

1 orange

Method:

Cook the cous cous according to the instructions on the package.

Heat a tablespoon of olive oil in a frying pan, and sear the scallops for a couple of minutes on each side until golden brown. Season with salt and pepper and cover and keep warm.

Use a vegetable peeler to finely slice the zest of the orange, and then cut with a sharp knife into thin strips.

Heat a little more oil in the pan, and add the zest and sugar snaps. Season and stir fry for a few minutes until the peas are heated through but still retain a little snap. Serve with six scallops and a spoonful of cous cous.

No-Stir Pea and Spinach Risotto:

You will need:

50g of unsalted butter

1 shallot or small onion, chopped

Salt and pepper

A small glass of dry white wine

750ml of vegetable or chicken broth

210g Arborio rice

A handful of frozen peas

2 handfuls of fresh spinach, rinsed well and chopped

25g of grated Parmesan

Method:

Preheat your oven to 180 degrees. In an oven proof dish (with a lid) over a medium gas or electric ring, melt the butter and gently saute the shallot with salt and pepper, stirring until soft. Do not allow it to catch.

Add the wine and let it bubble until reduced by at least half. Add the stock and Arborio rice, and turn up the heat until the mixture is boiling.

Cover the pot with the lid and transfer to oven. Cook for 20 to 25 minutes – the rice should be tender but still with a little bite remaining.

Add the peas, spinach and Parmesan, taste and season if required.

If the rice is undercooked and the risotto has become too thick, add a little water from a recently boiled kettle.

Courgette Pasta Bolognese:

You Will Need:

500g of lean steak mince or turkey mince

A good splash of olive oil

2 cloves of garlic, chopped

1 Large onion, chopped

2 carrots, peeled and cubed

4 courgettes, either cut with a spiraliser to make long strands or use a vegetable peeler to make fine strips.

150g of mushrooms, sliced – you can use button, white or chestnut

1 Tablespoon of tomato puree

2 x 400g cans of chopped or plum tomatoes

2 stock cubes, vegetable, chicken or beef

1 Tablespoon of soy sauce

Parmesan, to serve

A handful of basil leaves to serve (optional)

Method:

In a little olive oil, brown the mince until cooked through and broken into fine pieces. Set aside.

In the same pan, saute the onion until soften and translucent, then add the garlic, carrots and mushrooms and cook until the vegetables soften. Re-add the ince to the pan with the tomato puree and canned tomatoes. Fill one of the empty tomato cans with water and add that to the mixture, crumble over the stock cubes and bring to the boil. Cover, lower the heat and allow to simmer for one hour.

After an hour, add the soy sauce and taste to check for seasoning. Cook your spiralised or sliced courgettes in a little oil until they start to soften – do not overcook or they will become mushy. Spoon over the bolognese sauce and top with fresh basil and Parmesan to serve.

Hunter's Chicken:

You will Need:

4 chicken breasts, skinless

3 slices of proscuitto ham, chopped

1 tablespoons of olive oil

1 shallot or small onion, chopped

2 cloves of garlic, crushed

1 glass of dry white wine

1 x 400g can of chopped tomatoes

1 Tablespoon of tomato puree

250g of white or chestnut mushrooms, quartered

2 sprigs each of fresh sage, rosemary and flat-leaf parsley

Method:

In a large non-stick frying pan, cook the prosciutto in a little oil for a few minutes until it is crisp. Remove the ham and cook the garlic and herbs for a few minutes. Spread out the onions in the bottom of the pan and lay the chicken breasts on top. Season well and cook for a few minutes until the chicken and onions begin to brown. Remove the chicken breasts from the pan and set aside with the ham.

Add the canned tomatoes to the pan and stir to break them up. Add the wine and turn up the heat until the liquid starts to bubble. Turn the heat down and add the chicken and ham back to the pan. Add the mushrooms and a swig of water, then cover the pan and simmer for half an hour until the chicken is cooked through. Remove the lid and cook for a further 15 minutes until the sauce has thickened.

Chapter 5 – Exercise

Not only will exercise burn off calories, it will also tone your body, giving you a better shape. The more lean muscle your body carries, the greater its resting calorie demands will be – in other words, even when you aren't exercising, your body will still be burning more calories.

The benefits of exercise are manifold – it has been linked to better moods, a stronger immune system and higher energy levels. Everything about you will benefit from regular exercise – your skin, joints, mind and body.

There is no need to join an expensive gym and feel that exercise should be a chore. If you are not already a regular gym goer, think carefully before you sign up to one. Many people think that if they pay a monthly subscription, the thought of that money being wasted will somehow compel them to go. It will not. Before you sign up, set yourself a three week program of exercise that you can do at home. Plan to go for a run or a brisk walk, set yourself a number of sit ups and press ups to do every morning, and look on sites such as You Tube for exercise or dance routines for you to do in your living room. If, after three weeks, you have been able to stick to your plan, then you can go ahead and join a gym (you may even feel happy with your home-made regime and decide you do not require a gym membership) since you have shown that you have the discipline to make a gym membership worthwhile.

Some people enjoy group classes, such as dance, boxercise or pilates. Other people find that a solitary run can be a great way to relax and unwind. Find out for yourself what suits you personally.

You can also find ways to incorporate activity into your daily routine. Could you walk to work, walk to the shops, or out to meet friends? Rather than always meeting your friends for drinks or a meal, or to walk a film, why not suggest something more active? You could go for a walk, try a new exercise class or climb a tree together. You don't have to do the same thing every week or find the 'magic key' to weight loss – just look out for activities that require you to do a little more than sit down. What about an art gallery, museum or visiting a local landmark? Go swimming in a river (check to make sure it is safe first) or undertake a project around your home that requires physical activity. Playing sport is not the only kind of exercise that counts.

Conclusion

We hope you have enjoyed this guide to kick-starting your weight loss journey. After two weeks, you should start to see the benefits of eating more healthily and taking more exercise – not only with lower body fat and better muscle definition, but in a more positive outlook and increased energy. Every aspect of your life can benefit from increasing your general levels of fitness and eating a balanced, nutritious diet.

If weight loss is your goal, then it can be tempting to opt for quick-fix results and starve yourself in an attempt to get thinner quicker. However, a safe, sustainable level of weight loss is around 1 kg per week. This may not seem like a lot if you feel you have a large amount of weight to lose, but stick with it – just as important as losing weight is keeping it off. You will find it much easier to do this if you have made sustainable, long-term changes to your diet and exercise habits. Best of luck!